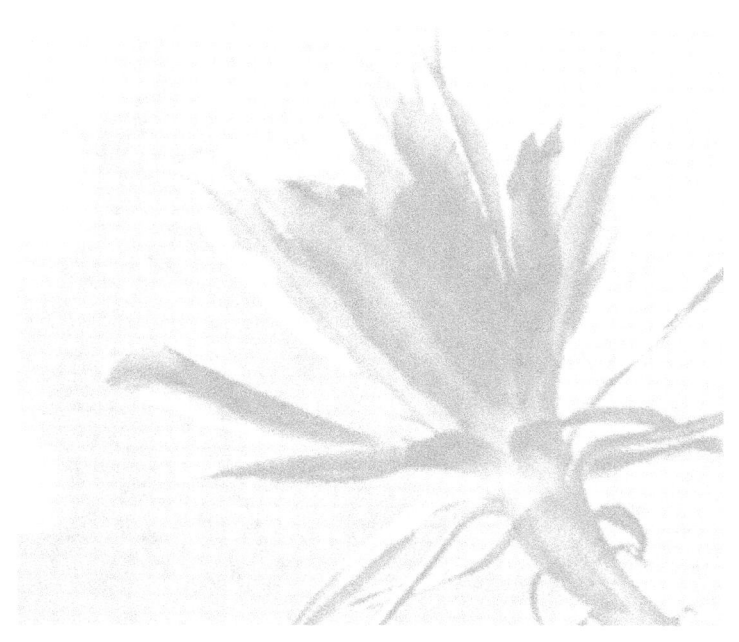

From Me to You

Inspiration to Live Well with Fibromyalgia

Cathryn Goodman, PhD

Second edition, 2012
First edition, 2008
Copyright © TXu1-283-450 2006

Published by
TFD Writing Services
PO Box 272
Glen Ellyn, IL 60138

Disclaimer

I am not an MD. I am not a nurse. This book is not endorsed by the Arthritis Foundation or any other medical group.

This is a personal letter from me to you; please treat it as nothing less and nothing more. It started out as an email to a friend of a friend and then morphed into something too big for an email.

I hope what I have to say can help you, but please make your own decisions concerning your health care with the help of the talented people in the healthcare profession.

Contents

About Me

I'm sitting in yet another physician's exam room; thankfully, this time I'm fully clothed. Although not an overly

I was diagnosed with fibromyalgia in 1997

modest person, I've come to despise white paper gowns with worthless plastic belts. Eventually, the doctor strides in—white coat immaculate, clipboard in hand, a smile pasted firmly on his face. He gives me a polite, disinterested "Hello, how are you?" and I tell my story one more time.

I recite a litany of aches and pains, treatments, and lack of results. This time I'm telling the story to a neurologist. After he does the usual "close your eyes and touch your nose" routine, he proclaims me neurologically sound. But in a parting remark, he mentions that my symptoms remind him of a lecture he attended the previous week on fibromyalgia. "Fibro-what?" I asked. He scribbled the word on the back of his business card and I began my journey to living well.

I was diagnosed with fibromyalgia in 1997 after 30 years of pain. In childhood, I was plagued by headaches and "growing pains." After a variety of brain scans and tests, my parents were told that there was something unusual about my brain wave patterns but no one had any idea what it meant.

I ended up on a cocktail of aspirin, caffeine, and Phenobarbital but the headaches and pain continued. Eventually I just stopped complaining. Still, I knew something was wrong. My recurring daydream was that a teacher would see my illness, pull me aside, and help me. It never happened. At night, I would lie in bed and wish that I wouldn't wake up.

As an adolescent, I sank into a deep depression but somehow kept putting one foot in front of the other. I buried myself in schoolwork and got good grades. I was teacher's pet and my parents were thrilled. Even my best friend had no idea how miserable I was.

In my early 20s I developed migraine headaches and chronic joint pain. The pain in my right shoulder from weight lifting remained even after arthroscopic surgery showed nothing was wrong. My right knee never recovered from overextending myself on a bike ride into a headwind. Lower back pain from lifting a box of books stayed for years.

Reactionary hypoglycemia (low blood sugar similar to a diabetic insulin shock) would send me into cold sweats and shakes without my knowing what hit me. My digestion was a mess, and by the age of 35, I couldn't sleep for more than two hours at a time. Walking and sitting were painful; depression and anxiety, pervasive.

Finally, after listening sympathetically to me for years, a friend recommended that I go the Mayo Clinic in Rochester, Minnesota for an exam. In desperation, I submitted a request for an appointment and described my symptoms on the registration form. After a few weeks, I was informed that my request had been forwarded to the neurology department. A few weeks after that, I received a denial for an appointment and was informed that I had been put on the two-year wait list for a general exam.

I was crushed. Knowing that I couldn't wait another two years for a diagnosis, I decided to find a local neurologist on the assumption that there had been some reason my case had been sent to that department. I picked a name from the phone book and made an appointment. That's how a card with the word "fibromyalgia" ended up in my pocket.

About You

If you have fibromyalgia, you've probably been suffering for years, too. You've probably been subjected to a battery of tests, all

> *You've probably been suffering for years, too*

of which turned out negative. Once you received the diagnosis, you may have spent years searching for a cure.

The bad news is that, for most of us anyway, there is no cure, no miracle medication, no one single thing that will fix everything. The good news is that you can still live well—differently but well. I know this from my own experience. I want to help you live well by sharing what worked for me.

The starting point for my recovery was the recognition that I needed to try everything I could get my hands on to fight fibromyalgia. I kept what worked and tossed out the rest. I think of it like panning for gold. I had to sift through a lot of worthless sand in order to collect enough nuggets of gold to make a living. It takes hard work and patience.

You can think of it like filling up a toolbox, tote bag, or backpack with strategies that will help you cope and move forward. Fill your bag until it overflows. Then you can pull from it, Mary Poppins style, when you need to.

My bag is full of ideas, from the sublime to the ridiculous; from pharmaceuticals to ice cream. I want to unpack my bag and tell you a story about everything in it. Take what you can from me and then go out and do your own collecting. Living well is a wonderful revenge and I know you can do it.

Doctors

As a girl, I read fairy tales. Even though my mother was a first generation women's libber, I bought the idea that men were

Become the CEO of your healthcare team

braver, stronger, and more capable than women. I knew I was weak and I thought a man would solve things. I found such a man and married him. He told me what to do, what to think, and how to act. He just about killed me. After 20 years with him, I realized I had to take care of myself. I wouldn't be able to do things perfectly, I would still lose my keys and be late for meetings, but I would be OK.

I had to learn the same lesson with my doctors. I started out thinking that I would find a doctor who would be my savior, my proverbial "knight in shining armor." He would be strong, intelligent, and attentive. He who would listen carefully, proclaim a diagnosis and prescribe an effective treatment program. I was angry and disillusioned when I found out that the fairy-tale hero isn't real.

Instead, I found that doctors are just like the rest of us—they come in all shapes, sizes, personalities, and approaches. And these days, many of them are women. Some are as arrogant as Zeus and won't bother to engage you in a conversation. Some will be baffled by your symptoms and give you a variation of the old adage: "Take two aspirin and <u>don't </u>call me in the morning." If you're really lucky, though, you may run into one or two who will team with you, and your other caregivers, to properly treat the whole you.

In the end, only you can take care of you. You have to take control of your health like a CEO takes control of a company.

Create a board of directors to give you their opinions and then make your own decisions.

My search for a health care team started with my internist and grew to include physical therapists, massage therapists, a pain management specialist, a rehab doctor, and a psychiatrist. I took something valuable

from each of them and put the ideas in my toolkit. Now that I've figured out how to manage my fibromyalgia, I just work with a general practitioner at a clinic in town. He is a good listener and is open to me being in charge of my treatment.

My recommendation is to try as many traditional and alternative health care providers as your time, money, and energy permit. I got the most help from a rheumatologist who specialized in fibromyalgia, but I learned from the other specialties as well. Keep trying new approaches until you have a good board of directors and you are firmly at the head of the table for your health care.

Resources

American Medical Association Doctor Finder
http://www.ama-assn.org/

American College of Rheumatology
http://www.rheumatology.org

Emotional Support

For most of us with fibromyalgia, depression goes hand-in-hand with pain. Does the chronic pain of fibromyalgia cause depression? Or does depression

Treat the physical and emotional pain

cause the chronic pain? I have had health care professionals explain it both ways. In some cases that might be true, but I think fibromyalgia is different. I knew a man who suffered cancer pain for years and he stayed optimistic. On the other hand, I had a female colleague who was chronically depressed but didn't develop physical pain.

It seems to me that whatever causes fibromyalgia causes both physical and emotional pain simultaneously—that's part of what makes it tough to treat. You need to treat both at the same time in order to live well. Plus you need to address other aspects of your lifestyle as well. In today's medical community it's hard to find a provider who understands this and is capable of providing it...hence the need for a board of directors that includes an MD and a therapist or psychiatrist.

My search for emotional support started as soon as I moved out of my parents' house. In college I saw a counselor-in-training at the university's medical center. That didn't last long, though, because she started to cry when I described my pain and depression. (I hope she got some help for herself, or perhaps changed professions.) In graduate school I tried again, and got some relief from a therapist at the local hospital. I continued counseling through the Employee Assistance Program of my first employer.

At present count, I've seen nine therapists. Some were helpful, some were not. Although they were all well-intentioned and compassionate, I never found a therapist who could eliminate the pain or the depression of fibromyalgia. Although it didn't help with the pain, my time in therapy did help me recognize and verbalize my feelings; feelings I had kept hidden from childhood. After a while, I could tell a story about my loneliness, shame and anxiety in a relatively detached manner. That created an environment in which I could move forward.

One of the biggest problems I had with therapists was leaving them. Even when it was clear that a therapist wasn't being helpful, it was very hard to end the therapy relationship because I had consciously built a sense of trust and dependence with him or her. Plus, I didn't want to hurt their feelings.

Breaking up has gotten easier over time, though. When I realized that I needed to be in charge of my treatment, I knew I had to be in charge of my relationship with therapists as well. Now I will interview a therapist before I sign on and I'm also prepared to say "Thank you, I've had enough" when the time comes. At this point I'm flying solo without a therapist. I still get depressed, but it's not as deep and not as dark as it used to be.

I urge you to be as deliberate and discerning about finding a therapist as you are in finding a doctor.

Resources

National Institute of Health
www.nlm.nih.gov/medlineplus/

National Alliance on Mental Illness
www.nami.org

Fire Your Therapist, Dr. Joe Siegler, MD

Antidepressant Medication

I fought antidepressant medication for a long time. Well, at least the ones I knew about. The first doctor I saw after my

> *Black-and-white turned Technicolor*

fibromyalgia diagnosis prescribed amitriptylene to help me sleep; it wasn't until I did my own research that I learned it was used treat depression. By then I realized it did help me sleep and that was a huge relief. Strangely enough, though it didn't ease my pain or depression. (It also had the very unpleasant side effect of giving me dry mouth which made it difficult to speak clearly. Later one of my docs switched me to trazadone and that helps me sleep without the dry mouth.)

Even after the trazadone, though, I refused to take Prozac or Zoloft or any other medication that I recognized as an anti-depressant. I think the biggest reason was the stigma of mental illness. I'm not really "crazy," am I? If I am, I sure don't want anyone else to know. Can I be fired for taking anti-depression medication? Can the courts take my kids away? To the last question, I was reassured by my attorney that any judge I faced would probably be on Prozac too!

Another strong deterrent was that my friends, relatives, and even Oprah told me that I could beat the pain and depression with a positive attitude. It's funny how healthy people think sickness is all in your head. As if we choose to be sick and depressed. As if we enjoy feeling like we want to jump off a cliff or hide under a rock. I tried thinking myself to wellness—I went to counseling, read books about thinking positive, and practiced meditation for years—I was still depressed and in pain.

I also thought that by treating the depression I would be treating a symptom, not the cause. If I got rid of the depression, wouldn't

I stop looking for the "cure"? What if something else was going on that I needed to figure out?

Plus, mind-changing drugs are scary. Would I still be myself if I took drugs? Was I betraying my real self by trying to be happy? Sure, I thought about throwing myself in front of a train just about every day, but I hadn't really done it, so I wasn't that bad off, was I?

What eventually turned me around was an MD who threatened not to treat me if I didn't take an antidepressant. I benefited from the rest of his treatment approach and wanted to stay, so I did as I was told.

Once I finally took the meds, it was like Dorothy leaving Kansas—my black-and-white world turned Technicolor. The weight that bent me over like Quasimodo lifted and I walked upright. "Is this what everyone else feels like?" I wondered. "This is awesome!" In retrospect, all I did by resisting medication was waste a lot of time being miserable that could have been spent living well.

The drugs were amazing but not a cure; I didn't instantly become an optimistic person and I'm still not. I didn't become strong and athletic and I'm still not. What the medication did, however, was lift enough of the anxiety, depression, and pain for me to use the other tools effectively. I still had plenty of work to do but it was a huge leap forward.

The drugs didn't take work immediately either; it took a few weeks for me to get the full effect. In the meantime, I was uncomfortably sleepy and thirsty. Your body is probably going to take a while to adjust, too. Be patient. I know how hard it is, but be patient. Give yourself a couple of weeks to get used to a drug and then decide if it is going to help.

Eventually, as you are released from the worst of the depression and find other coping strategies, you may be able to decrease the amount of medication you need to stay functional. I take significantly less than the normal dose for "major depression" to get the benefits. Taking more doesn't improve my condition significantly and that's part of the reason that I think fibromyalgia is something different from "pain caused by depression" as I mentioned in the section about emotional support.

For me, it didn't matter what brand of antidepressant I took, they all worked equally well **if I was also taking** trazodone. Trazodone or Zoloft by itself does nothing for me. I think that is worth repeating because so many people get discouraged when an anti-depressant doesn't help them—in order for me to live well, I need to take a tricyclic anti-depressant like amitriptilyne or trazodone **and** a selective serotonin re-uptake inhibitor like paroxetine.

For you, it may make a difference which drug you use. Keep trying until you find the medication—and the dose—that works for you. A word of caution, though: weaning off one medication before starting another can be a nightmare. See if your doc will allow you to switch directly from one to the other as you make comparisons.

Resources

"Antidepressant Medicines; A Guide for Adults with Depression," U.S. National Library of Medicine, National Institutes of Health http://www.ncbi.nlm.nih.gov/pubmedhealth/PMH0004898/

Pain Medication

I had the same attitude about pain medication that I had about antidepressants; I didn't want to take them. I wanted to tough it

I wasted a lot of time being in pain

out. I admire people who can boast, "I've never taken an aspirin in my life;" they sound strong and capable, just the way I want to be. And again, I think I wasted a lot time in pain.

I also had "pain amnesia." It's similar to what they say about giving birth: It's a good thing you forget how bad it is or you would never have a second child. For me, when the pain went away I would think it was gone for good. "Aha," I thought, "I'm cured." Wrong. It was just a temporary reprieve. The pain always comes back.

I never did take narcotics for the pain—I never had a doctor take my pain seriously enough to prescribe them—and I think that's probably a good thing. I've heard from other patients that oxycodone, morphine, and others aren't a long-term solution and, of course, have bad side effects. I did find, however, that analgesics like ibuprofen, aspirin, and acetaminophen are helpful **if** I'm taking the antidepressants and I'm using all of the other strategies in this booklet.

Now, I take an analgesic (ibuprofen, aspirin, acetaminophen) at the first hint of pain. If I don't, it just gets worse. I had one doc tell me to take a pill before I started cleaning house. I thought he was nuts. Taking medication when I didn't need it? My mother would have had a fit. But, mother aside, it turns out he was right for my fibromyalgia. Take a pill before you pull out the vacuum instead of after and you may keep yourself out of bed with back pain. Just don't tell mom about it.

Of course, there are risks to this approach and you'll have to keep track of what you're doing. For example, I've taken so much of one type of over-the-counter painkiller that I'm allergic to it. Now I take a different type and I'm not sure how long that's going to last. There's also a concern since these drugs can irritate your stomach and damage your liver. Discuss this with your health care professional, but I urge you not to let the concerns force you to live with chronic pain.

If your story is different from mine and you already take pain medication without relief, work on some other strategies. Don't be discouraged, though. Remember, you're going to need a lot of tools in your toolbox to cope effectively with fibromyalgia.

Physical Therapy

Drugs and medications probably aren't going to be enough to get you feeling well again... Add a physical therapist to your team—

> *Some did more harm than good*

a physical therapist who understands fibromyalgia, that is. The first physical therapists (PTs) I saw at first were associated with orthopedic surgeons. They were used to treating professional athletes and weekend warriors with sports rehab programs.

These folks, as well-intentioned as they were, did me more harm than good because I didn't respond to therapy the way their other patients did. They would put weights in my hand and wonder why I couldn't lift increasingly heavier weights. "Yesterday you lifted two pounds," they would say. "Today you should do five." They didn't know that lifting two hadn't made me any stronger and that five would be intolerable. We were all discouraged.

Another problem was that they were used to treating one painful spot at a time. At one point I was sent to physical therapy for my knee. The therapist said, "Lie down on your side and do 15 leg lifts."

"I can't lie on my side because my shoulder is too painful," I responded.

She raised an eyebrow and said, "It says on your chart you're here for knee pain."

"Yes," I said, "but my shoulder hurts too."

Silence.

She had no idea what to do so I quit going. Just like a talk therapist, be prepared to walk out on a physical therapist if he or she isn't helpful or does anything that causes you more pain.

After lots of bad experiences, I ended up with some PTs who were effective for me. They were European trained and started treating everyone at their "core" starting with back and abdominal exercises. Only then would they start to work on the other problem areas. I ended up with an exercise that helps minimize the pain in my back, another to help my shoulder and some great stretching routines.

In order to keep my lower back, upper back, and shoulder relatively pain-free, I need to stretch and exercise every day. It's guaranteed that if I get lazy and stop, I'll have more trouble. Fortunately, I also know that when the pain comes back, I don't panic. The hard part is maintaining the discipline to exercise when I feel good.

I recommend that you shop for a PT just like you do for an MD and a talk therapist. Fill your toolbox with exercises as well.

Resources

If you can't find a physical therapist in your area who understands fibromyalgia, you might find this book helpful. The knee exercises have worked well for me. Available at Amazon.com

Pain Free: A Revolutionary Method for Stopping Chronic Pain, by Pete Egoscue and Roger Gittines

Hypoglycemia

I have reactionary hypoglycemia, which means that if I eat too much sugar, my body produces too much insulin and sends itself into self-induced insulin shock

The test for hypoglycemia nearly killed me

with shakiness and cold sweats. Physically, it's the same as when a diabetic overcompensates for food intake with too much insulin. Even though my body makes too much insulin instead of too little, I need to eat like a diabetic to live well. That means frequent small meals with balanced protein, fat, and complex carbohydrates.

I had pretty much figured this out on my own, but my GP had read that hypoglycemia was associated with fibromyalgia and thought it would be useful as a diagnostic tool—especially since he had precious little else to go on for a diagnosis. The test for hypoglycemia nearly killed me, though, and I share my story as a cautionary tale.

The test involved having me drink a bottle of orange syrup and then measuring my blood sugar every hour for six hours. Since I didn't want to take a day off work for this, we arranged do the test on a Saturday morning. Everything was fine for the first couple of hours. By the third hour the doc went home for the day, and it was just me and nurses. By the fourth hour my blood sugar had started to drop and I was feeling faint. They discontinued the test at five hours when my blood sugar dropped precipitously to 30 and I went into convulsions. The nurses were completely unprepared for the reaction, they had assumed that I was diabetic, and they had dug into their purses for a candy bar to give me.

Needless to say, if you suspect that you have hypoglycemia, be careful about the test. Bring a high-carb snack with you and have someone available to drive you home to a big meal.

Resources

This site has an interactive program to help you plan your meals to balance blood sugar.
http://www.nlm.nih.gov/medlineplus/tutorials/diabetesmealpl anning/htm/index.htm

Headaches

When I was at my worst, I had a migraine headache several times each month. I had the typical stabbing pain over one eye that would migrate to the top of my

Ibuprofen, coffee, and chocolate

head and my neck. Sound and light would cause my head to throb. I would get sick to my stomach. Fortunately for me, I could still get through a day at work and the most important chores at home. But, I was miserable. I tried a couple of the prescription migraine drugs and used them as directed, but they didn't help.

What I did find helpful is the max dose of ibuprofen with a coffee chaser (I got the idea from an expensive over the counter migraine pill). If I stay on this, the headaches and nausea will clear up in a couple of days. Take the over-the-counter, non-prescription drugs if they work for you, or develop your own combination with coffee, chocolate, and pain killers.

I've found that many times my migraines are triggered by tension in my upper back and neck. Massage therapists are great at working out the knots and releasing the tension. You may find that as the other strategies take effect, you'll have fewer migraines, too. Now I only get a migraine a few times a year.

Research released in April, 2007 suggests that migraine headaches are accompanied by undetected brain damage. This may lead to treatment protocols that target the source of the problem, not just the pain. It's too early to tell for sure what's going on, but you might want to talk to your doctor about it.

Cardiovascular Exercise

I was never an athlete. In fact, I was the proverbial "last one picked for basketball." In my early 20s, though, I ran, swam,

Walk, don't run
Walk, don't sit

and lifted weights regularly. Fibromyalgia eventually forced me to give it all up. The running made my right knee ache and the swimming aggravated my left shoulder that I hurt with the weight lifting.

Now, I walk. I make time to walk 20 to 30 minutes a day, a few times a week. At the beginning, this was very difficult. What helped the most was having a sympathetic friend at work; he would walk with me every afternoon at break time. He would walk as slowly as I needed but would push me, very gently, to go a bit farther every day. By the end of a couple of years, I could walk two miles and go up five flights of stairs.

That might sound pathetic to your athletic friends or spouse or your own inner voice. "Walking is for wimps," they might say. "What you really need to do is run, ski, bike, [fill in the blank]."

Easy for them to say, they don't have fibromyalgia. Don't let them talk you out of gentle exercise. Do what you can without making yourself feel worse. Take it easy.

Walk, don't run, but walk don't sit.

Once you've got the worst of the fibromyalgia under control, find an exercise strategy that works for you. It will clear your head, give you energy, and help you feel alive again.

Supplements

Vitamin D, minerals, oils, extracts, herbs, spices, shark cartilage, magnesium injections, Co-Q 10, Asian remedies, homeopathic, and on and on— I've tried them all.

None of them reduced my pain

None of them reduced my pain, even if I took them for months.

Even though supplements didn't work for me, you will need to come to your own conclusions. When you're in the grip of fibromyalgia, I wouldn't want to talk you out of trying anything.

The best approach might be to try pharmaceuticals first to get yourself functional and then try the alternative approaches to see if you can wean yourself off the meds.

Allergies

Before my diagnosis with fibromyalgia, I thought my headaches and stomach problems could be from allergies. After my diagnosis, I thought the fibromyalgia might be caused by food allergies.

> *I eliminated wheat and dairy for six months*

First, I went to an MD who tested me for acute reactions with a skin test. He was looking for allergens that would create rashes or respiratory problems. Yes, in fact, I was allergic to dust, dust mites, mold, cats, and dogs, just like a whole lot of other folks who don't have fibromyalgia. I made a valiant effort to eliminate them with mattress covers, filters over the air vents, and air purifiers. None of them lessoned my pain or depression.

Another health care practitioner assumed that I was allergic to wheat and dairy. I eliminated wheat and dairy from my diet for six months. I was still in unbearable pain and depressed.

Later, I saw a chiropractor who recommended a blood test for chronic reactions to allergens. My GP drew the blood, stored it properly, and sent it to the lab. I tested positive for peppers, swordfish, brazil nuts, yeast, and a chemical used in farming. In response, I drank only filtered water and I didn't eat any of these foods for six months. Once more, I didn't see any effect on my pain or depression.

I would recommend getting tested for allergies, just in case, but keep working on your other strategies. I don't think it makes sense to torture yourself with a difficult dietary plan if it doesn't get you a significant improvement.

Thyroid Problems

This is another one that some people like to claim is at the root of the problem for fibromyalgia patients and yes, hypothyroidism does share many symptoms with

Each new doctor tested my thyroid level

fibromyalgia including fatigue, exhaustion, digestive issues, depression, and some degree of muscle and joint pain.

Each new doctor I saw tested for this as part of the routine before considering other options. My thyroid level is smack in the middle of normal and I got really tired of this being blamed for my condition.

That said, thyroid problems are treatable, so it makes sense to get tested for this early in your search for a diagnosis and treatment. And if you do have a thyroid problem, that doesn't mean you don't also have fibromyalgia. Keep looking for other strategies until you are feeling truly well.

Resources

A description of hypothyroidism can be found on the Mayo Clinic website:
http://www.mayoclinic.com/health/hypothyroidism/DS00353

Track Your Pain

My education is in engineering so I'm used to solving problems with numbers and calculations and spreadsheets. Before my diagnosis with fibromyalgia, I

I kept an Excel spreadsheet of my pain

kept an Excel spreadsheet of my pain with a rating from 1 to 10 each day. I would print out the graphs and take them to my G.P.

"See," I would say, "This is how miserable I've been."

It didn't have much of an impact on him, but I felt it justified my complaints.

Tracking my pain also gave me some sense of control—something that seems to go out the window with fibromyalgia. It seemed that pain would come and go without cause. By tracking my pain, I at least had something I could look at.

After my diagnosis, several of the pain management seminars I attended also recommended keeping a pain diary. Try making a daily sheet and enter how you feel physically and mentally in the morning, at noon, and at night. Make a note of what is happening and what you are trying to do to make yourself feel better. Look for triggers (lack of sleep, the noisy neighbors, etc.) and for relief strategies (a nap, earplugs, or a call to the cops to report a disturbance).

I think it's also important, though, to understand that it is not your fault if you are in pain. No matter how well you control what you do, no matter how positive you try to think, you may not be able to cure yourself of the pain and depression. You may still need medication and a counselor and a physical therapist. Don't be too hard on yourself. Do what it takes to live well.

Slings and Things

One of the difficulties with
fibromyalgia is that I look healthy
even when I'm in extreme pain. If
you break a leg, people can see
the cast, open doors for you, and

> *We look healthy even*
> *when we are in pain*

give you some much needed sympathy. If you have a raging
fever, your face will flush, you'll break into a sweat and someone
will tell you to go home and get to bed. But if your shoulder is
painful from fibromyalgia, other than the grimace on your face,
there are no outward signs of the very real pain that you feel on
the inside.

Because I looked healthy, I always felt embarrassed asking for
help. I imagined people would think I was lazy and I'm sure
some of them did. But after a while the pain wore me down, and
I knew that I needed help; I simply was not going to get through
even the simplest chores by myself.

To make it easier for me to ask for help, and easier for others to
give it, I made my pain visible. If I had pain in my shoulders, I put
on an elbow sling. For my knee, I put on a knee brace. For my
back, I would carry a cane. You get the idea. The props gave me a
socially acceptable reason to ask the checkout person at the
grocery store to help me get the groceries to the car.

Why not make your pain visible? If you don't already have a
collection of slings and things, you can probably find them at
your local pharmacy or grocery store

Resources

Walgreens carries medical supplies on its internet site:
www.walgreens.com

Moving

For me, fibromyalgia meant that even the smallest tasks were unbearably painful. I couldn't put the dishes away, carry a bag of groceries, or lift my one-year-old

> *Even the smallest tasks can be painful*

son. When I felt pain, I thought I was causing myself more injury and I wanted to stay motionless.

The demands of my family didn't go away, though, and I had to find different, less painful, ways to get the most necessary of my chores done. I read about ergonomics, listened to my health care team, and developed some strategies. Here are a few of them for you to consider.

Around the house

- Instead of reaching up to a shelf in the kitchen cabinet, use a stepstool. Get a stool that is light enough to nudge across the floor with your foot since you probably don't feel like bending over to carry it.
- Place items at the edges of counters and desks. If you're still able to work, arrange the times at your desk in a semicircle the size of your arm's reach. Stand up to get the less-used items at the back.

Grocery shopping

- Make frequent trips with lighter loads
- Ask the clerk to fill your bags half full and take them into the house one at a time. It takes forever, but it's worth it—and a little extra walking is good if you can handle it.

Laundry

o Transfer wet clothes from the washing machine to the dryer one piece at a time; wet jeans are a killer.

o If your back is a problem and you have a top loading washing machine, reach into the machine while holding your back straight. Here's how: put one hand on the edge of the machine to keep your balance, lift one leg out behind you and bend from the hip. Sounds weird? Think of how golfers pick up their ball. They hold onto the putter, kick one leg back, bend from the hip, and reach down. Same idea.

At a sink

o Rest one foot on something when standing at the bathroom or kitchen sink to take pressure off your back. Some people recommend that you open the cabinet under the sink and rest your foot there. I've never had a cabinet where I could do that without banging my knees. What works better for me is to have another light stool nearby.

Restricting your range of motion will probably be necessary when you are feeling the worst of the fibromyalgia. It will help you get the pain under control and use some of the other strategies effectively. But once the worst is over, try to get moving again. In the long run, that's going to be the best strategy to avoid further injury and pain.

To help keep your body from getting too tight while you are being careful about how you move, make sure to do the stretches your physical therapist gives you. And keep stretching, even after you feel better.

As the pain recedes, challenge yourself to move out of your safety zone. Cautiously start to reach out and stretch your arms and torso. Try taking two stairs at a time. If something starts to hurt, back off and wait a while. But keep trying. Remember, the goal is to live well again, not just to keep living.

Resources

The Arthritis Helpbook has a lot of great strategies. It's available from the Arthritis Foundation website and Target.com

The Arthritis Helpbook, by Kate Lorig and James Fries

Sitting

It's not fair, but even sitting and lying down can be painful with fibromyalgia. Here are some strategies that might make resting more restful.

> *Sitting and lying down can be painful*

First, I always sit with a small pillow to support my lower back. I've found that it is important to keep my back in a neutral position. That is, an inward curve at the neck and lower back. Have you seen one of those plastic skeletons hanging in your doctor's office or on TV? Think about what the back looks like; it's curved in and out instead of straight or rounded. Try to keep yourself looking that way, even though it is tempting to slouch.

For the car, I purchased a seat frame that is adjustable to the curve of my back and that keeps my seat from sinking down into the cushion. I found it at medical supply store; you may have to hunt to find one. You'll also need a helpful and strong person to bend it until it's tailored to the right position.

At home, I avoid soft couches and choose a firm, but not hard, chair. I always have a small pillow handy for my lower back and sit up straight. (By the way, if you're sitting at home watching TV or reading, remember to get up and stretch regularly. I need to get up every half hour or so. Set a timer to remind yourself if you need it.

Going out to restaurants or the theater where you can't control the seating can be an ordeal. The worst chairs are the ones with an opening in the lower back just where you need the support most. When I was in the most pain, I purchased a smaller version of the car seat and took it with me to a concert, movie, or conference to be prepared for open-back chairs. Pride took a back seat to comfort. At one concert, another patron turned to me and said "Hey, that's not fair! My back is killing me. Wish I had one of those!"...Ha, revenge!

When I was better, I could manage by taking a sweater with me and folding it into a cushion for my back. If you're the fanny-pack type, you can fill a small pack with a soft pillow or sweater and keep it at your waist. When you sit down, push it in back and you've got an instant support pillow. That also works well if you tend to forget your pillow or sweater in the seat when you get up to leave. I've lost quite a few sweaters and sweatshirts that way.

If you're working, arrange your chair, keyboard, and monitor so that your feet are supported, your back is in a neutral position, and your neck is in neutral. Use a footstool, chair cushion, or monitor stand to get everything in position.

Resources

You can purchase the Sacro-Ease seat from this site:

http://www.mccartys.com

Sleeping

I went at least ten years without getting a good night's sleep. I would wake up every two hours or so and have to get up and move around. If I wasn't actually

I spent 10 years without a good night's sleep

in pain, I was just uncomfortable. My legs would get jumpy and restless and I would toss and turn. My husband banished me to the couch in the living room—not an ideal solution for my back pain or my marriage.

I never thought of asking a doctor about this problem. Lots of people have insomnia, right? Once I found a doctor that knew about fibromyalgia, though, he got me on the tryciclic anti-depressant and I could finally sleep through the night. Once again, it wasn't a cure for all of the symptoms, but it is an important step in the right direction.

Even with the medication you might find that getting comfortable in bed is just as challenging as sitting, but the principle is the same: Keep the S-shape in your back and keep your spine from twisting. I find it most comfortable to lie on my side with a thin pillow under my head and another between my knees. This keeps my neck straight and prevents my top leg from twisting my back forward. These days they make full-body pillows which look fabulous. If you've got the cash, a thermo-molding pillow can be very comfortable too, particularly for back sleepers.

If you sleep with someone else, I suggest that you consider getting yourself a separate bed. Like Ricki and Lucy, you may find that two beds are better than one. If your partner snores, consider sleeping in a separate bedroom. Romance has its place, but it's great to have your own bed just for sleeping.

Limitations

There are some things that, no
matter how careful I am, still
cause me pain or discomfort. If
I'm feeling really bad, I just don't
do them. If I'm feeling better, I

*Recognize your
limitations*

may decide to do them anyway and deal with the pain. Mostly, I
try to limit how much I do of the painful things.

For example, I need a regular sleep schedule. When the
fibromyalgia is in full force, I need a good ten hours and I can't
stay up past 10 p.m. I need to say "no" to invitations for a late
movie or party because driving home late with restless legs will
make me crazy. It's just not worth it, so I go to the early show
whenever possible. If there's a late show that I really want to see,
or when it's New Year's Eve, the only thing to do is to be
prepared and try not to scream too loudly on the drive home.
(I've found it really distracts the driver.) As I've gotten better,
I've been able to loosen up on this restriction, but know I'll be
achy for days if I stay up too late.

When I travel, I try to keep my sleep on my home time zone. I
live in the Midwest, and if I travel to Washington, D.C., I turn in
early instead of going out with the gang for dinner and drinks. If
I'm in California, I get up early and work in my room until the
breakfast meeting starts. International travel is completely off
limits. In my former corporate position, that limited my career
climb. Now that I've given up on the corporate ladder, it doesn't
make much difference. At one point, though, I turned down an
invitation to a wedding on the Rhine River to avoid the pain of a
long flight, jet lag, and messed-up sleep schedule. C'est la vie.

Speaking of work, I also can't sit glued to the computer for hours
at a time. I need to stretch every half hour or so, and every
couple of hours I need to get up and walk away. I can get so

caught up in my head that it literally cramps my body. I take a walk around the building, sit in the cafeteria and people watch, or stop by a buddy's cube and chat for a minute or two.

I also can't do physical activities for very long. Even if the garden is overgrown with weeds, I can only pull them for five minutes at a time. I remind myself that they'll still be there tomorrow. And I can only vacuum one room and clean one part of the kitchen floor at a time.

I used to get frustrated and angry about my limitations. Now I realize that this is all a part of who I am. If it's who you are too, it's OK to scream and yell for a while. Then settle down and figure out your own balance between what you can and can't do. As a wonderful pain management coach once reminded a group of us, "You're living in the desert now. Enjoy the cactus and forget about the willow trees."

Things You Love

I think it's important to focus people, places, and things you love. I spent most of my life isolated from other people because of my pain and

> *Focus on people, places, and things you love*

depression. In the past few years, as some of the weight of fibromyalgia has lifted, I've found that I am a much more social person than I thought I was. I have developed a wonderful circle of friends from my work, church, and neighborhood. I love spending time with them in low-key casual situations (early in the evening with a back cushion and good chair!).

Perhaps you have a hobby that you can still enjoy. If you can't run anymore, can you walk? If you love to cook, can you bake a delicious desert instead of a seven-course meal? If you love animals but don't have the energy to care for one, try volunteering to work a few hours at an animal shelter. If you love movies but can't sit still for two hours, sit in the back of the theater so you can get up and stretch every 20 minutes or so.

If you can afford it, buy yourself fresh flowers and enjoy them every day. Get someone to help you put up a bird feeder and watch the birds enjoy the feast. Spend time with the grandchildren, or nieces and nephews, and leave when they start to get on your nerves. If you've got your own kids and they drive you nuts, get a sitter on a regular basis so you can get out by yourself.

Do whatever gets you out of yourself and brings you a moment of joy. I think the chemicals that your body produces in these moments can help counteract the fibromyalgia. Spend some time and energy seeking out these moments and relish them.

Do What Feels Good

Do what feels good and do as much of it as you can. For someone healthy, that might be an invitation to hedonism, but if you've got fibromyalgia, it is simply a survival strategy.

Simply a survival strategy

My favorite indulgence is a good massage. I get a massage from a professional as often as I can afford to. I always let the therapist know that I have fibromyalgia so he or she can take special care. If that's not an option, perhaps you and a friend could a massage class so you can get a free back rub every day!

On a smaller scale, get a facial or a scalp massage when you get a haircut. (Avoid the shampoo, however, because leaning back in beauty salon shampoo chairs is a killer.) Some manicurists will give you a hand massage that feels wonderful too.

Get a makeover at the cosmetic counter in a department store; it feels good to be pampered for a little while. Soak in a hot bath or join a club with a whirlpool. If you have the means, install a whirlpool in your home.

Fragrance can be powerful for unlocking feelings of joy. Use scented candles that make you feel warm and cozy. Bake a batch of chocolate chip cookies. Just don't eat too much or you'll feel guilty and that will ruin the whole thing. Take the cookies to your family or friends instead!

Spirituality and Religion

The depression and pain of fibromyalgia created in me a deep-seated self-pity. I saw happy people around me—friends, parents, co-workers—and I resented their pain-free lives. I felt separate, different and alone. However, once I took medication and learned to exercise appropriately and started sleeping better, once I started to peak my head above the fog, I realized that everyone has some kind of problem they carry with them. Even the happy ones.

I realized that there are no pain-free lives. Whether it is the illness of a parent, the loss of a job, betrayal by a loved one, a child's dangerous behavior, or one's own pain, everyone has a burden to bear. Some handle their burdens well, some don't.

This revelation released the chains of my own selfishness and allowed me to feel the joy of compassion for others. It brought me a sense of belonging to a community, of something bigger than myself.

The ancient Indian/Buddhist parable of the woman and the mustard seed illustrates my point. It was told to me in one of my pain management workshops. My interpretation, roughly based on the original, goes like this...

***

A young man and woman meet, fall deeply in love, and marry. Soon the young woman becomes pregnant. The husband and wife make joyful plans for the baby and the life they will have as a family.

Before the baby is born, the father is called off to war and within weeks he is killed in battle. The young woman is grief-stricken; her only solace is the baby that is growing inside her.

In time, the baby is born and she rejoices in its presence. One night, the young woman falls asleep with the baby in her arms. When she awakens, she finds the baby still and cool; it is no longer breathing.

She jumps from her chair with the little body in her arms, wraps it in a blanket, and runs to find the physician. He opens his door to find the frantic woman clutching a bundle wrapped in a blanket.

"Please, please," she cries. "Help me wake my baby!"

The doctor pulls the blanket away from the little face and says, "I am so sorry, my dear, your baby is dead, there is nothing I can do for him."

"Then I will find someone who can," she screams, turning on her heel and running to the apothecary shop.

"Please, please," she cries, "Give me medicine to wake my baby."

The chemist peers under the blanket and repeats the doctor's words, "I am so sorry, your baby is dead and there is nothing I can do for him."

The little body is now cold and gray but she screams even more loudly and runs to the home of a wise woman who lives in the hills nearby.

"Please, please," she cries, "I need a prayer to wake my baby. He is all I have in this world."

"I understand your grief and sadness," she replies. "I will help you *if* you can return to me with a handful of mustard seed from a household that has never grieved the death of a loved one."

"Thank you!" the young woman cries. She races back down the hill and knocks on the first door she finds.

"Can you spare me a handful of mustard seed to save my son," she asks.

"Of course," the occupant says and retrieves seeds from the kitchen.

The young woman takes the handful of tiny seeds and starts to leave, but then turns back and asks, "Have you known the grief of death in this house?"

"Yes, two months ago my father died after a long illness. I think of him each day when I see his empty bed."

The young woman returns the seeds to the occupant and rushes to the next house and the next and the next. It is the same at each house in the village.

"Yes, my husband was killed by wolves."

"Yes, my son was slain in battle."

"Yes, my father was executed."

"Yes, my sister drowned herself."

"Yes, my brother was killed in the mines."

"Yes, my daughter was stillborn."

Finally, the young woman falls to the ground and sobs, "My son is dead and I am all alone."

She trudges back to the hut of the wise woman and says, "I am ready to bury the body of my son."

"Did anyone give you mustard seed?"

"Yes," answered the young woman, "many people gave me mustard seed but each had grieved the death of a loved one. It was selfish of me to ask you to bring my baby back from the dead."

"Then you are not alone in your sorrow," the wise woman states.

"I am not alone," realizes the young woman and she stands up a little straighter.

"What will you do now?" the wise woman asks.

"I will return to the village and help with the other children," she replies. "They are all my family now."

***

I have come to believe that a belief in something larger than our own selfish selves is necessary to live well. The "something larger" can take many forms. For many people, it is a belief in a wise and powerful monotheistic God. Others visualize the higher power as a life force or energy. For some, a connection with the grandeur of nature gives a sense of belonging and awe. For others, it is found in love and compassion for humanity itself.

Resources
Find a Catholic Church
http://www.parishesonline.com/scripts/default.asp

Find an Evangelical Christian Church
http://www.efca.org

Find a Synagogue
http://www.uscj.org/Find_a_Synagogue_Sea5425.html

Find a Humanist Society
http://www.americanhumanist.org/what_we_do/local_groups

Don't know which church is right for you? Try this:
http://www.beliefnet.com/story/76/story_7665_1.html

Be Impatient. Be Patient.

At first, having been trained as scientist, I wanted to try one treatment at a time to determine its effectiveness. I wanted to take medication A for a while to see if it helped. Then I wanted to try medication B and compare the effects. Then I would add physical therapy and drop the meds to see what happened. It turned out to be a frustrating approach. I never got better and I still couldn't figure out why.

After years of failure with that approach, I hit rock bottom and was willing to try anything and everything. I took the antidepressants and the pain medication. I got acupuncture, massage, and physical therapy. I saw a psychiatrist and a counselor. With this approach, I started to find relief.

When you're miserable, be impatient. Hit the fibromyalgia fast and hard with everything you can. Then, when you've got the symptoms down to a tolerable level, slow down, and pick and choose what works best for you.

But now, finally, I can be patient with my pain. When it flares up, I don't panic. Hallelujah! When my knee gets sore, I know the medication and walking will help it feel better. When my shoulder starts burning, I have a message therapist you can work out the kinks in my back. I know that the pain killers, the antidepressants, and the physical therapy are going to get this thing under control again. I know I've got something in my bag that will do the trick. While I'm equally confident that it will come back again, it is a wonderful feeling to know it will go away for a while too.

Putting it All Together

I hope you feel inspired to become CEO of your health care team! Pack your bag with exercises, medication, distractions, and things you love. Living well with fibromyalgia is hard work but the reward is tremendous!

Below is a list of what I need to do to live well. Don't let it scare you; once you get into a routine it's not that overwhelming. Don't think I'm perfect either; I get lazy and there have been months at a time when I haven't followed my own advice. When I get feeling too crummy I'll pull out the list again and get back to work. Most important, don't take this list as a prescription. It works for me but you will have to find what works for you.

- paroxetine in the morning for the pain and depression
- ibuprofen before strenuous activities and for flare-ups
- daily 10-minute stretching and strengthening exercises
- daily 30-minute walks
- daily 5-minute meditation/relaxation exercise
- daily 30-minutes of a hobby (gardening, sewing, reading)
- Hourly stretching when I'm doing desk/computer work
- trazodone in the evening to help me sleep
- 8-10 hours of sleep each night on a regular schedule
- meals with balanced protein/fat/carbohydrates
- avoidance of yeast-containing foods
- monthly massages
- minimized interaction with critical/mean/harsh people

Keep trying, you can feel healthy, happy, safe, and strong—perhaps for the first time in your life. I know it!

This booklet has been about what works for me. I would love to hear what works for you. Send me an email and I'll post your success story on my web page.

Acknowledgements

Many people have helped me live well. I want to thank Linda for leading me to Mayo Clinic, Mark for getting me walking, Soni for letting me make her guest room my home, Thomas for teaching me the superman exercise, Jerry Ann for showing me the flowers in the desert, Dr. Z for pulling a diagnosis out of thin air, and James for making me laugh. Thanks also to the unknown writers of "ER" who showed me what my life would become if I didn't take charge.